Because...
Someone I Love Has Cancer

Kids' Activity Book

American Cancer Society

Published by the
American Cancer Society
Health Promotions
250 Williams Street NW
Atlanta, Georgia 30303-1002

Copyright ©2003 American Cancer Society
All rights reserved. Without limiting the rights under copyright reserved above, no part of this publication may be reproduced, stored in or introduced into a retrieval system, or transmitted in any form or by any means (electronic, mechanical, photocopying, recording, or otherwise), without the prior written permission of the publisher.

Printed in China
Designed and illustrated by Shock Design, Inc.
Cover designed by Shock Design, Inc.

5   4   3   2   09   10   11   12   13

Originally published in 2003. Reprinted in 2009.

A Note to the Reader
The information contained in this book is not intended as medical advice and should not be relied upon as a substitute for talking with your doctor. This information may not address all possible actions, precautions, side effects, or interactions. All matters regarding your health require the supervision of a medical doctor who is familiar with your medical needs. For more information, contact your American Cancer Society at **800-227-2345** (**cancer.org**).

EDITORIAL REVIEW
Terri Ades, M.S., A.P.R.N.-B.C., A.O.C.N.

MANAGING EDITOR
Gianna Marsella, M.A.

EDITOR
Amy Brittain

BOOK PUBLISHING MANAGER
Candace Magee

SENIOR LEAD, CONTENT
Chuck Westbrook

CONTRIBUTORS
Karen Dorshimer-Chaplin, M.Div.
Sue P. Heiney, Ph.D., R.N., C.S., F.A.A.N.
Janice Haines
Marge Heegaard, M.S., A.T.R., L.I.C.S.W.
Heather Higginbotham
Suzie McKenzie
Lisa R. Murray, A.T.R.-B.C.
Sharon Schweiker
Anneke Smith

For more information about cancer, contact your American Cancer Society at **800-227-2345** or on the Web at **cancer.org**.

Quantity discounts on bulk purchases of this book are available. Book excerpts can also be created to fit specific needs. For information, please contact the American Cancer Society, Health Promotions Publishing, 250 Williams Street NW, Atlanta, GA 30303-1002, or send an e-mail to **trade.sales@cancer.org**.

For special sales, contact us at trade.sales@cancer.org

Note to Parents and Other Caregivers

THIS BOOK IS FOR CHILDREN WHOSE LOVED ONE HAS CANCER. Children faced with the uncertainty of cancer may have many thoughts and feelings about it. For parents and caregivers, helping children sort through the range of feelings during this time can be a challenge.

Parents often struggle with what to tell their children when there is a diagnosis of cancer in the family. How much they need to know and can handle depends on the children's ages and coping skills. However, talking with them about cancer is essential. In doing so, children learn that their families are there for support. It also helps them know that they can count on the people they love and trust to be honest.

One of the first steps toward helping children cope when a loved one has cancer is talking about it—before, during, and after treatment. The second step is to help them develop the tools for coping with their feelings and reactions. This book is designed to help children between the ages of six and twelve recognize their feelings and develop coping skills to help them deal with cancer in the family.

How Do Children React?

School-aged children may act sad by the news of a cancer diagnosis. They may also be angry, scared, or grumpy. Children often worry that cancer is contagious. They know they can "catch" a cold by being near someone who is sick, so it makes sense for them to be confused. It may be helpful to explain that cancer is not like the flu, but is a different kind of illness. It is also common for children to think something they said or did caused the cancer. They can be reassured by statements such as,

"Nothing you did caused the cancer. None of us had anything to do with causing it."

Although children at this age are widening their circle of friends and adults, there is still a strong need for security and routine. But it may be hard to keep up a normal routine. Children may feel that their lives are out of control. They may also become frustrated, or simply act silly and behave younger than they really are. This often occurs in children who are under stress. For example, a child may become clingy, return to security objects (such as a teddy bear or blanket), or wet the bed at night.

When children have changes in routine, their negative reactions are usually temporary. Providing as much comfort and reassurance as possible is generally enough to help them feel secure. These behaviors are usually short-lived and usually go away as long as they know they will be cared for.

Children are often unable to express directly how they are feeling in words. It is easiest for them to show and explain their feelings through activities such as playing, puppets, painting, and drawing. Older children might prefer writing poetry or stories, or drawing. This book is intended to help children understand their feelings and learn to use their creative skills to cope.

How Is Art a Healing Tool?

What, in particular, do children express in drawings and stories? Themselves, first and foremost—how they look, what they do, and how they feel. They also show how they are related to others and to their world. The activities in this book use drawings and stories to allow children to express their feelings in pictures and words.

Art is one of the oldest and most natural forms for a child (and humankind, for that matter) to express ideas and feelings. It is created in many forms: drawings, sculpture, dance, stories, and so on. As a healing tool, art allows ideas, thoughts, and feelings to escape onto the medium. And in the case of drawing, emotions flow onto paper. There is no "right" way for someone to draw a picture, write a story, or mold a figure. Each piece of art is personal because every child has unique abilities and insights.

When art is used as a healing tool, experts recommend that parents, caregivers, or other trusted adults ask children open-ended questions about their drawings such as, "What is this a drawing of?" For example, if a girl draws a picture of a small girl, ask her, "What's going on in the picture with the little girl?" While explaining about the little girl, she may actually reveal things about herself. Children often give details about a drawing when, in fact, the picture applies to them. More questions about what is going on in the drawing can be asked from the information they provide.

Who Can Benefit from This Activity Book?

Although this book is designed for children between the ages of six and twelve, it may also be helpful to older or younger children. Younger children may need someone, such as an older sibling, to read the instructions. But since most of the activities involve drawing, younger children can do them without help. Older children may be encouraged to complete the activities with a sense of fun. And they may even learn a few things about themselves along the way!

Because some children may be more likely to share their drawings (and feelings) while working on or after completing a page, you may wish to let your children know that you are not far away as they work in their book.

What Is the Best Way to Use This Book?

Because this book may stir up a lot of different feelings, you may wish to browse through the activities first. If you have concerns about using the book with your child, talk to a mental health professional at your treatment center. This might be a social worker, psychologist, nurse counselor, or chaplain.

What Can I Tell My Child about Using This Book?

You may wish to give this activity book to your child in a special way. You can explain that the activities can help him or her understand, think about, and talk about what it is like when a loved one has cancer. Emphasize to your child that this book belongs only to him or her. Tell your child that the book can be kept private or shared with someone else.

A suggestion for telling your child about this activity book is to say, "In your book, it's okay to color, draw, or write anything in any way you want to. No one else will look at your book unless you say so."

If this activity book is being used in a setting outside the home, such as in a support group, it may be helpful to tell children that they are not being graded, and they will not be forced to share anything they don't want to.

Tips for Sharing

This book is meant to be a private place for children to express themselves. But you may gently encourage your child to share thoughts and feelings that it brings up. You might use some of these questions or comments to talk with your child:

- What is your favorite activity? I'd like to see it, if you are willing.
- What is the hardest activity you have done? What was hard about it?
- What was easiest activity you did? What was easy about it?
- If you met another child whose parent has cancer, what would you tell him or her about the book?
- I am always here to talk with you about your book.
- I won't look in your book, but I'd like to know your thoughts and feelings. I hope you will feel comfortable to share them with me.
- Don't worry about me. I might be sad or happy when you tell me how you feel, but all kinds of feelings are okay.
- How do you feel today?

What Is in This Activity Book?

This book contains six sections. A brief description of each section is provided below. Each is designed to focus on helping children deal with a loved one's illness and the crisis of cancer. The hope is that as children work through the activities, they will become more able to cope with their concerns about cancer.

1 *Things Change*

Children at this age can grasp the concept of change, but may not be able to deal with it well, especially when it affects their daily routine. The first activity uses a simple metaphor like the seasons changing to show that things around us grow and change. This section continues with other activities related to changes that occur because of the illness and ends with an activity that asks the child to identify a positive change that has come out of a diagnosis of cancer.

2 *Label Your Feelings*

An activity with faces and feelings lets children associate emotions with appearances. Taking this a step further, the feeling thermometer visually encourages children to identify their feelings at the time.

3 *Know Yourself*

This section encourages children to explore their feelings in more depth. Understanding how and why we feel a certain way is sometimes difficult, even for adults. But we grow stronger if we understand how we feel and why we feel that way. Part of this understanding involves knowing what causes a feeling and where the feeling comes from, which the activities in this section address. Children who have a loved one with cancer can learn to realize that sad feelings are strong right now because a loved one is sick.

4 *Boost Your Self-Esteem*

Maintaining healthy self-esteem in school-aged children during a diagnosis of cancer in the family can be difficult with all the changes that are happening. The activities in this section offer some ways to help build self-esteem.

Children who have healthy self-esteem possess some or all of the following "senses":
- a sense of safety (including family self-esteem)
- a sense of belonging—being a part of the group, which includes the family and groups outside of the home
- a sense of personal pride and ability—solving problems on their own, being creative, and knowing what to expect
- a sense of trust—being able to trust and be trusted
- a sense of responsibility—doing things without being watched or checked up on
- a sense of making real choices and decisions
- a sense of support and reward—earning and receiving positive feedback and praise
- a sense of accepting mistakes and failures

5 *Find Your Strengths*

For children, coping can come in many forms. Two ways of coping are thinking about the future in a positive way and talking to family members and friends about worries. The activities in this section are intended to help children find their strengths. This helps them feel more in control rather than acting out, becoming depressed, or feeling anxious. Activities include a chart for helping around the house, an outline of the child's hand with unique character traits identified, and a list of things the child excels at doing.

6 *You Can Handle It*

Rather than distracting children from difficult feelings (creating diversions), these activities focus on looking to the future, drawing and writing about encouragement and support, and using the imagination to regain balance and a sense of control.

The family and group activities (in the next section), in addition to the activity book, also help children develop coping skills.

Additional Information and Resources

The activities in this book are based on clinical experience from experts and feedback from parents and children. A variety of professionals in the field were consulted to gain strategies and insight into what helps children cope and even grow from the crisis of cancer in the family.

This book should not be used as a substitute for professional services. Always seek the advice of your doctor or other qualified health professional with any questions or concerns you may have about a medical condition, including mental health issues. If you feel your loved ones and/or children would benefit from further help, hospital social workers, nurses, psychologists, clergy members, and school counselors are good resources to ask about support groups in your area.

If you notice any significant changes in behavior that last for more than a couple of weeks, these are **warning signs** that a child is having difficulty. Seek help from a mental health professional immediately.

For more information about how to talk with children about cancer and a list of suggested reading materials for caregivers and children, contact your American Cancer Society at **800-227-2345** (**cancer.org**). You may also contact the Society to order a copy of the book *Cancer in the Family: Helping Children Cope with a Parent's Illness* or other books of interest.

For your convenience, these pages have been perforated so that you may remove this section and the next before you give the book to your child.

Family and Group Activities

Why Do These Activities?

The activities in this section provide an opportunity for sharing and spending time together. This could be one-on-one with a child and a family member, within a counseling group, or among family members and friends. Group activities can be healthy for children because they are engaged with people with whom they feel comfortable. These activities have been designed to help the family (or other group) solve problems before they become overwhelming. They can help relieve tension by bringing concerns out in the open. Talking about problems may even make them easier to manage.

You can use these activities to learn about how your children think and feel about cancer, as well as other things that are going on. It is healthy to express difficult emotions through talking, drawing, and playing. Perhaps you will have a better understanding of your children's mental health and coping abilities by their behavior, conversation, and creations.

When Is a Good Time to Do These Activities?

Setting up a regular time for activities involving the whole family or counseling group can be a good strategy. You may also choose to do an activity at the end of scheduled family meetings. Some of the activities are appropriate for a child and an older sibling, a parent, or family friend. They have been designed so that children and trusted others can talk about their thoughts and feelings about cancer in their lives.

Activities

Many of the following activities allow for candid discussions with children about their artwork or creative projects. Open-ended questions that are neutral and without judgment can lead to very telling responses from children. Simple acceptance without any assumptions often allows children to freely share their thoughts and feelings.

For some of the following activities, extra materials, such as scissors, glue, scrap materials, magazines, and so on, may be required. Use these activities according to your needs and situation.

(Note: "Child" or "group" may also refer to a group member or a number of children and vice versa.)

- ***Find stories about other people*** who have had cancer and read them with your child.

- ***Explain what will be happening*** to the loved one with cancer by using a doll. You can also use dolls for other members of your family or group. With younger children, role play. Children often express what they are really feeling in their play, as well as using dialogue for their dolls.

- ***Gather a stack of old magazines, scissors, and glue.*** Create a "feeling collage" together by using meaningful pictures from the magazines. After the collage is finished, talk with your child about what it means.

- ***Plant a small garden with your child.*** Use a variety of things in which to start the seeds, such as milk cartons, seed starters, or egg cartons. Poke several small holes in the bottom of the container for drainage. Add potting soil. Have your child gently plant the seeds in the soil and water so the seeds don't wash out. Be sure to get seeds that germinate easily and do not require special care such as rye seeds. Place the container in a window or another spot that gets a lot of sunlight. Sit back and watch them grow! Use the garden as a metaphor to discuss what is happening with the loved one with cancer.

- ***Have clay, blocks, and other creative materials to use*** to work out feelings that you and your child have. (Clay is especially good to work out frustration.) Or make play dough and encourage the child to sculpt or create a feeling. To make the play dough: Combine 2 cups flour, 1 cup salt, 1 tablespoon cream of tartar, 2 tablespoons oil, and 1 cup water with food coloring added. Cook all ingredients over low heat, stirring constantly until dough pulls away from the sides of the pan and forms a lumpy mass. Remove from heat, cool, and knead the dough. Store in a plastic bag or plastic container in the refrigerator.

- ***Plan for laughter by presenting a comedy show.*** Be creative with the format, such as taking turns telling a joke, or writing and acting out a skit. Remember: Laughter is good medicine.

- ***As a group, create a strong box*** (like a safe that holds money). You can use a pencil box, purchased box, gift box, or shoebox. Encourage your child to decorate the outside of the box by using collage, coloring, or painting. Use white school glue for the collage, or use tacky glue to add objects (like a seashell to represent that he or she is a good swimmer). Tell the group (or child) to place pictures of things that remind them of their strengths on the box. You can tell the group that their strengths help with coping.

    After the outside of the box is done, tell the group that the inside of the box is for their feelings. They may want to cut words from a magazine, or draw or write words that express their feelings and paste them on the inside of the box.

    Now get them to talk about the inside and outside of their boxes. For the outside, you might help them relate what strength can help them deal with specific stresses. For example, being a good student might help one get information about a loved one's illness.

    For the inside of the box, teach the group about feelings. Tell them that all feelings are normal, and some feelings are hard to have. Placing them in the box helps the feelings to be less powerful. Let them know they can continue to add feelings by writing on a piece of paper and placing it in the box. Encourage them to come to you when they want to talk about feelings or have a strong feeling that bothers them.

- ***As a group, make a video or slide show*** (by using pictures converted to slides on a computer) about what the experience of cancer in the family has been like for them. Or, suggest that they perform a play to show how they felt throughout treatment. You can see how they "play" different people in their lives and how they relate to you and to each other.

- ***Buy a large piece of poster board and write a special saying on it*** (or use the slogan your child created – see page 37) with a magic marker in large letters. Then cut the board into seven pieces and have your child put the pieces together. You can also purchase blank puzzles at hobby or craft stores.

- ***Create a "healing space"*** (such as a bulletin board or shelf) in your house or classroom to represent that healing continues even after treatment is over. In this place, you might ask every participant to find and leave a symbol of healing. For example, a stone might be for strength (because it's rock hard). You might place a family picture or a picture of yourself. Suggest adding some objects such as fall leaves for their beauty. Children might bring things home from school or from a walk in the yard. Looking at this place can help you and your children center and focus on being relaxed. You can add objects to your healing place at any time so that it becomes an ongoing project.

- ***Explain to the group how to play charades.*** Create cards with actions on them. Taking turns, each person picks a charade card and acts out the emotion or action on the card. In addition to "Pretend someone stole all the money from your piggy bank" or "Pretend it's your last day of the school year," include cards with actions related to the cancer experience. This might include "Act out how you felt when you first learned about the cancer" and "Pretend you are a doctor in a hospital."

- ***Helping your family or group write, tell, or draw stories*** about your times together can be healing for all of you, as well as become a future memento. An easy way to do this is to make a scrapbook, journal, or memory album. You might choose to focus on a special activity that you did with each child.

- ***Make a family tree book*** and tell about the people in your family. Allow the child to pick out pictures and make his or her own picture book of memories. Another suggestion is to collect baby and recent pictures of group members. Discuss common traits among family members and how each person has changed. (This activity also highlights the concept of change.)

- ***A similar activity is the "Family Tree."*** Decorate a tree with the things that make your family or group special. You might also wish to buy a small potted tree on which to hang symbols of hope. Or, you can use branches from the ground outside and put them in a can with dirt and small rocks to hold the branches in place. Hang notes with messages written on them, ribbons, hearts, or other special tokens and reminders of hope.

- ***Reading stories together that focus on feelings can be very healing for children.*** Young children enjoy *I Am So Mad* by Mercer Mayer. Older children can read aloud from fantasy stories such as *The Neverending Story* by Michael Ende or *The Chronicles of Narnia* by C. S. Lewis. Stories are great because they indirectly show ways of sharing feelings and coping. Discuss the themes and messages of each book after reading them.

- ***Another activity that requires less energy is to tell shared stories.*** You might begin with "Remember when we..." and let the child fill in the blanks. Each of you can share favorite memories. You can also use a tape recorder so your child will have a permanent record.

- ***A similar activity to the one above is to allow the child to ask the person with cancer about his or her childhood.*** How was it different from the child's childhood? How was it similar? Encourage the child to draw pictures based on the stories. (This is something they can do together quietly.)

- *Make a mobile.* Have your child write words for feelings he or she is having right now on the different pieces of paper or cardboard. Then let the child color the pieces and attach them to a wire clothes hanger with string or yarn. Discuss the many mixed emotions that can come about at a time like this and how, like feelings, the mobile changes and moves at different times.

- ***Just as a real clock tells time, the Feeling Clock tells feelings.*** Allow the group to list as many feelings as they can, as someone records the feelings named. Using a large circle (or a paper plate), divide the circle into as many areas as feelings listed. Each child may create a Feeling Clock, or the group can create one. Allow the child to color each of the areas labeled with a feeling on the clock. Next, draw and cut out an arrow. Attach the arrow to the clock with a small metal fastener. Now ask each child to point the arrow to the feeling that he or she has right now about the person with cancer. How would the child like to feel in the future? Tell the group to use the clock to let people know how they are feeling. You can mount the clock(s) on a family bulletin board or even the refrigerator.

- ***As a family or group, create a Welcome Home sign*** for the loved one with cancer returning home from the hospital. (You may ask the child if you can use his or her design on page 79.)

- ***To emphasize the concept of change, play a game of matching change cards*** (similar to "Memory"). Create the cards by cutting cardboard pieces of the same size and using pictures from magazines or original drawings. Card pairs might include a caterpillar and a butterfly, summer and winter, sun and moon, and so on. Allow the child, family, or group to suggest matching pairs.

- ***Instruct each person to make a fingerprint on paper.*** The child then labels whose it is and asks each person, "How do you feel about your loved one being sick?" (This activity can further explain that everyone has different feelings, just like they have different fingerprints.)

- ***Create a Trouble Monster by using a paper plate.*** On the plate, cut a wide, open mouth. Allow the child to create the face of the monster. Staple or tape a paper bag behind the mouth. Troubles written on pieces of paper are placed in the mouth.

- ***Make an encouragement box*** by using a shoebox with a drop slot for words of reward, encouragement, or coupons (see Helping Out Coupon on page 63).

- ***Design and create a group flag*** with inexpensive material and scrap pieces. Be sure to hang your flag high!

- ***Every family has rules,*** and each family member has special jobs. Using everyone's input, make a list of your Family Rules. Cut it out, and place it on the refrigerator. Be sure to recognize those who follow the rules and do their assigned chores.

- ***For families, set aside Family Night,*** where each family member takes turns planning dinner and an activity for the whole family. Children learn planning and responsibility, as well as respect for the person who regularly performs these tasks.

- ***Play the Talking Game.*** Create cards that encourage conversation. Questions might range from "What age would you like to be and why?" and "What animal would you like to be?" to more serious questions like "Do you think it is ever all right to tell a lie?" Make the questions appropriate for the ages of the group. Place the questions in a box and have each person pick a card and respond to the question. This game can be played at dinnertime, during Family Night, or at special times set aside for talking. Here are some suggestions for card questions related to cancer:

> *How did you feel when you first found out about the diagnosis of cancer?*
> *I wish that I . . .*
> *What do you worry about the most?*
> *What do you say when you tell others about cancer?*
> *Who or what could you NOT get along without?*
> *What do you like most about yourself?*

- ***Create and design a Family or Group Shield.*** Cut cardboard or poster board into the shape of a shield. Decorate the outside of the shield with a slogan, drawings, pictures from magazines, and/or photos that represent the group or family. On the inside of the shield, have each member of the group write his or her name. Discuss how the things that represent the group can help in coping with cancer.

- ***Make your own family portrait.*** Obtain a picture of each family member (or individual in the group) by using a Polaroid camera, digital camera, recent photo, or drawing. As a group or family, draw a background or setting, such as a favorite vacation site, the home, or other place. Have each group or family member place his or her picture on the setting. This activity encourages family unity and teamwork. Ask questions about the portrait, such as why someone placed his or her picture in a certain place.

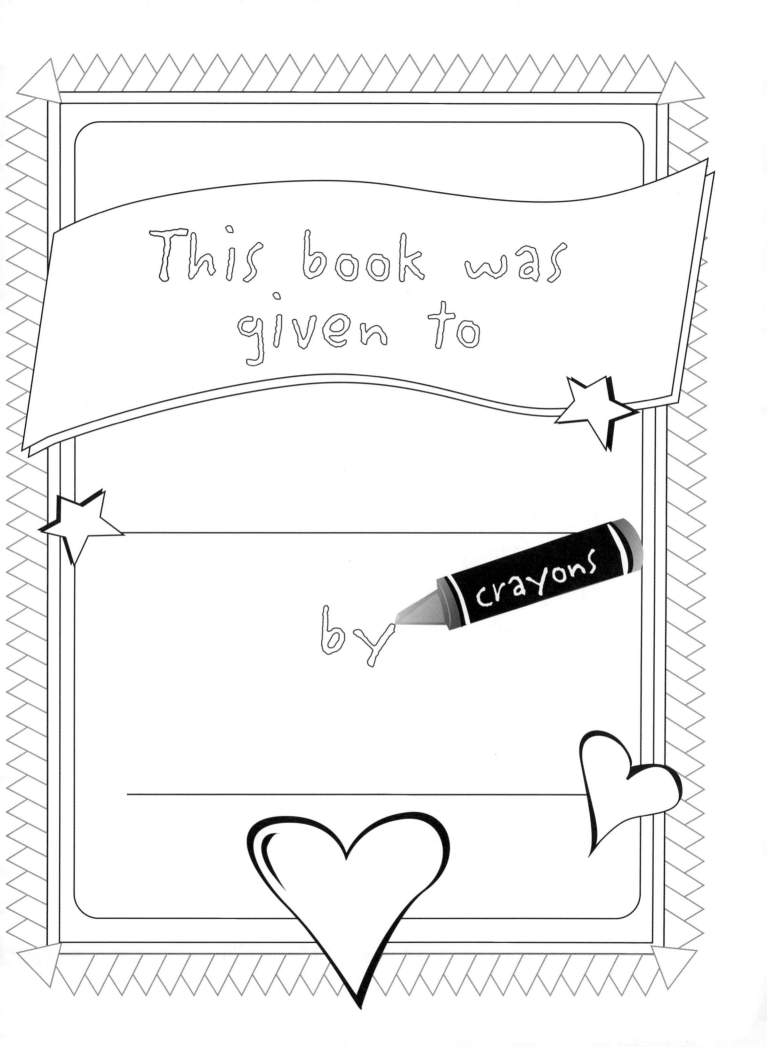

About Your Book

This book will help you understand and talk about what it is like when someone you love has cancer. It belongs to you—

and only you!

You can choose to keep your book to yourself so that no one else will look at it unless you say it's okay. Or you can share your book with someone you trust. Sharing might help you feel better.

Do only a few pages at a time. You can skip any exercises you want. If you get worried or sad after doing an activity, talk to someone you trust. Take a break and come back to your book another time.

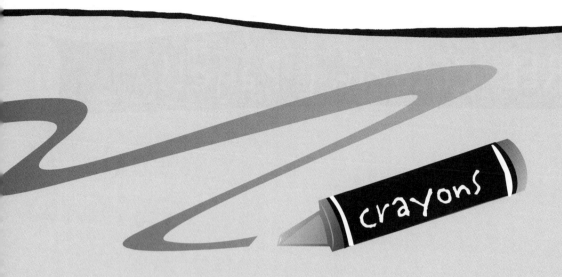

You are not being graded.

This is your book, so it's okay to color outside the lines and use the book the way you want.

Most of all, be creative and have fun!

Maybe you will learn some things about yourself!

FREE Coloring Page!!

©2003 American Cancer Society. All rights reserved. Copies of this page may be reproduced only for personal, educational, and/or noncommercial use by the reader.

Things Change

Everything changes. For example, you get older and taller every year. Even though things change, there are people you can count on.

Someone you love has cancer. But you hope your special person will get well again.

This part of your book will help you understand that cancer changes some things in your life.

Seasons Change

Changes in nature happen all the time. The seasons change too. Draw a picture of each season.

Fall	Winter
Spring	Summer

Changes in My Home

Things may have changed in your home or family since the person you love got cancer. What has changed? Has any room in your house changed a lot? Mark the rooms that are different and explain what has changed.

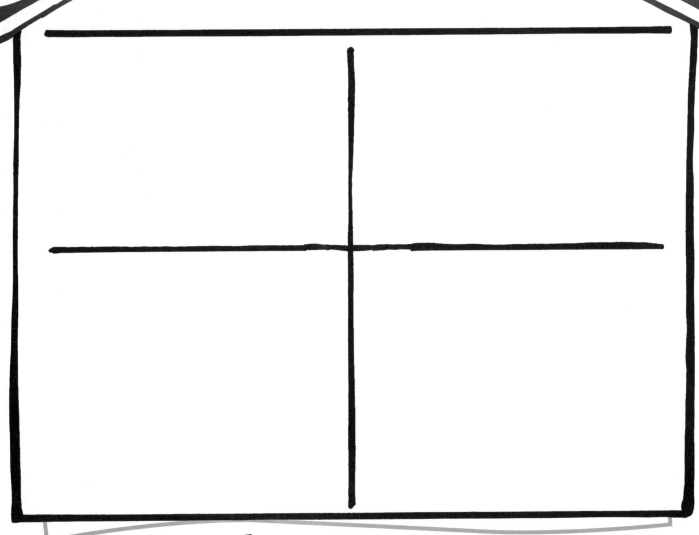

Before

Draw a picture to the left side of the door that shows what it was like before cancer.

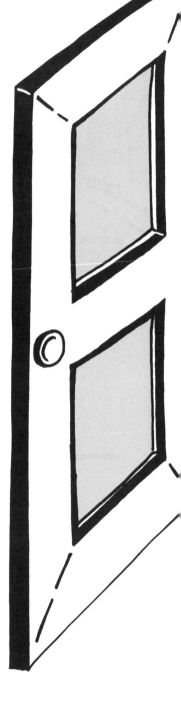

and After

On the right side of the door, draw what it is like after cancer.

People Get Sick

Sometimes a person's health changes because of an illness like cancer. Draw or write about the person you love who has cancer.

Create a Hat

Radiation (*ray dee AY shun*) and chemotherapy (*key mo THER uh pee*) are ways that cancer can be treated to make it go away. In some people with cancer, these treatments can make them lose their hair. Create a hat for the person you love who has cancer.

I Still Have Questions

Maybe you still have questions about cancer. Write or draw them in the space below. You may want to ask someone you trust about your questions.

Not All Change Is Bad

Maybe cancer has helped you to care more about someone or something. Draw a picture of a good change that cancer has brought to your family.

FREE Coloring Page!!

LABEL YOUR FEELINGS

All feelings are okay. Some common feelings are anger, sadness, happiness, and fear. Some feelings are harder to have than others, such as when you're scared or sad. You might feel this way because someone you love has cancer. If you feel really down, talk to an adult you trust. It will help you feel better.

This part of your book will help you to understand how you are feeling.

Name the Feeling Face

Write a feeling that goes with the picture.

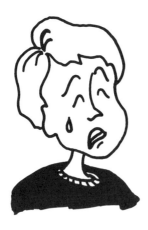
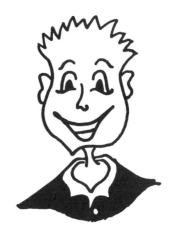
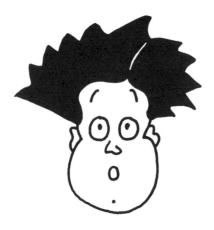
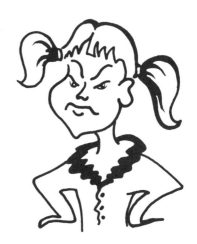

Draw your own Feeling Face and name it.

Feeling Thermometer

How are you feeling today? Color as high or low as you feel.

I'm Great! —

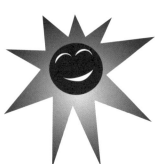

Okay. —

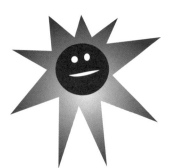

So-so. —

I'm really down. —

If you're feeling down or worried about the person you love who has cancer, draw a picture or write about someone you can talk to.

Feelings and My Body

We know about feelings by how our bodies react, such as having cold hands when we are nervous or afraid. Color or label the parts of the body where you notice feelings in your body.

Pick Yourself Up

Make a list or draw something that you can do to help yourself feel better when you feel sad.

Open Hearts

Sometimes it can make you feel better to talk about your feelings. In the hearts, write names, draw, or paste pictures of the people you can share your feelings with.

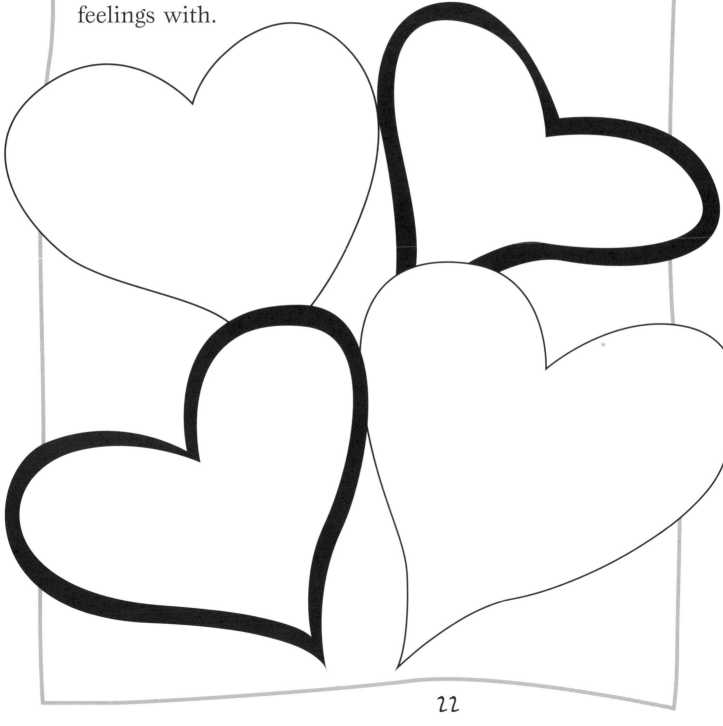

Know Yourself

You will feel better if you learn to understand some things about yourself, like how you feel, what you think, and how you act.

This part of your book will help you understand your feelings. It will also show how feelings, actions, and thoughts are related to each other.

My Feeling Faces

This is how I look when I am:

mad

sad

scared

worried

happy

Now choose another feeling. Draw a feeling face for that feeling.

Thoughts and Feelings

Write or draw how you felt:

How did you feel when you first found out that the person you love has cancer?

What makes you feel sad about the person you love who has cancer?

What do you like most about your family?

What is the worst part about the person you love being sick?

My Checklist

When someone you love is sick, you may have all sorts of thoughts and feelings. Put a check in the box that relates to how you think or feel.

	Always	Sometimes	Never
It's okay to cry.	☐	☐	☐
I should hide my feelings so that I don't bother anyone.	☐	☐	☐
It's wrong to be angry.	☐	☐	☐
Worry affects how I sleep.	☐	☐	☐
I feel like I can't do anything right.	☐	☐	☐
I think something I did caused the cancer.	☐	☐	☐
It's okay if I don't want to talk about my feelings.	☐	☐	☐
Nobody cares about me anymore.	☐	☐	☐
I'm afraid that someone else I love will get cancer.	☐	☐	☐

©2003 American Cancer Society. All rights reserved. Copies of this page may be reproduced only for personal, educational, and/or noncommercial use by the reader.

I've Been Sick, Too

Sometimes the medicines used to stop cancer from growing can make people feel sick. Draw a picture or write a story about how you feel when you are sick.

E-mail Pals

Pretend you just got an e-mail from your friend who is far away. Write a letter or draw a picture to tell your friend how things are going.

| Send | Save | Delete | Address Book |

To:
Subject:

How Does It Make Me Feel?

Draw a picture or write a story about what it's like when someone you love has cancer.

Fill in the Blanks

Write what you think and feel about cancer, or the person you love who has cancer, to complete the sentences below.

I don't see _____ as much.

_____ is more tired than before.

We don't _____ anymore.

I often feel _____
_____.

I used to _____ before cancer.

I worry more about _____
_____.

The worst thing about cancer is _____

_____

_____.

I miss _____ the most.

I like to _____ more now.

Sometimes I have to take care of _____

_____.

_____ is different now.

FREE Coloring Page!!

©2003 American Cancer Society. All rights reserved. Copies of this page may be reproduced only for personal, educational, and/or noncommercial use by the reader.

Boost Your Self-Esteem

Sometimes worries make us feel bad about ourselves. But we are all special. Self-esteem is a word that means how you feel about who you are and what you can do.

This part of your book will help you feel better about yourself.

Snowflakes

No two snowflakes are the same. No two people are the same. Write or draw something about you that makes you special.

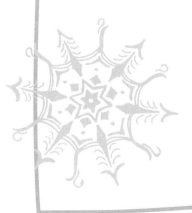

T-Shirt Message

Think about how people put messages or catchy slogans on T-shirts. A good slogan is short and powerful. Decorate this T-shirt with your family's slogan.

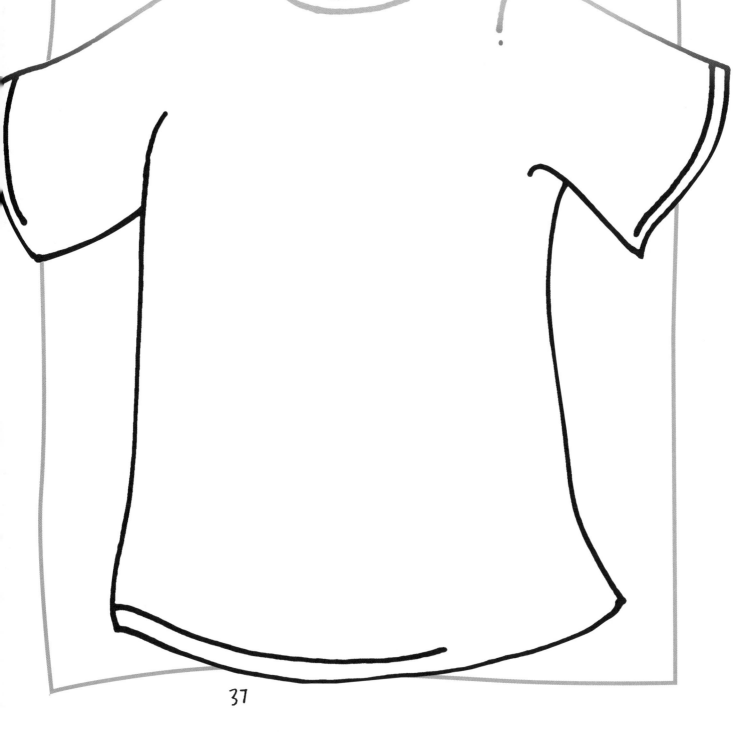

What Would You Say?

What would you tell someone your age who just found out that someone he or she cares about has cancer? Write or draw about it.

Favorite Toy

Here is a picture of my favorite toy.

I like it because _____

_____

_____ .

What's Your Favorite...?

What's your favorite song or poem?

_____

Write some of the words of the song or copy a verse from a poem that you like best.

Draw a picture of how this song or poem makes you feel.

Best Friends Are Great

My best friend's name is _____.

Draw a picture or write a story about you and your best friend.

Why is he or she your best friend?

What do you like to do together?

All Grown Up

Write a story and draw a picture of what you want to do when you grow up.

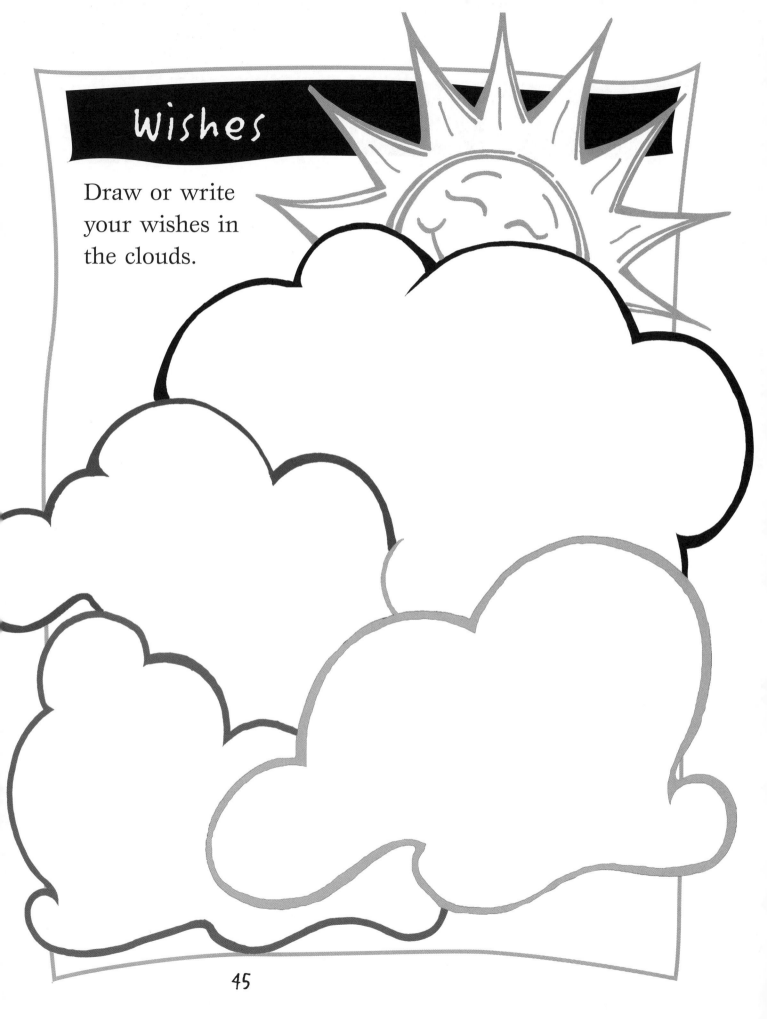

FREE Coloring Page!!

©2003 American Cancer Society. All rights reserved. Copies of this page may be reproduced only for personal, educational, and/or noncommercial use by the reader.

Find Your Strengths

Some people are really good at spelling. Others are better in math, baseball, or drawing. Something you are good at doing is called a strength.

This part of your book will help you think about and show your strengths.

Fill in the Blanks

I know I can _____

_____

_____ .

I am proud that I _____

_____

_____ .

I am really good at _____

_____ .

Dad or Mom is pleased when I _____

_____ .

A good idea I had was _____

_____

_____ .

A nice thing that someone said to me was _____

_____

_____ .

©2003 American Cancer Society. All rights reserved. Copies of this page may be reproduced only for personal, educational, and/or noncommercial use by the reader.

On My Own

I can do a lot of things by myself. Here's a picture, story, or poem about something I can do on my own.

Good Habits

You can have good habits to help you stay healthy. Circle the things you do that can help you stay healthy.

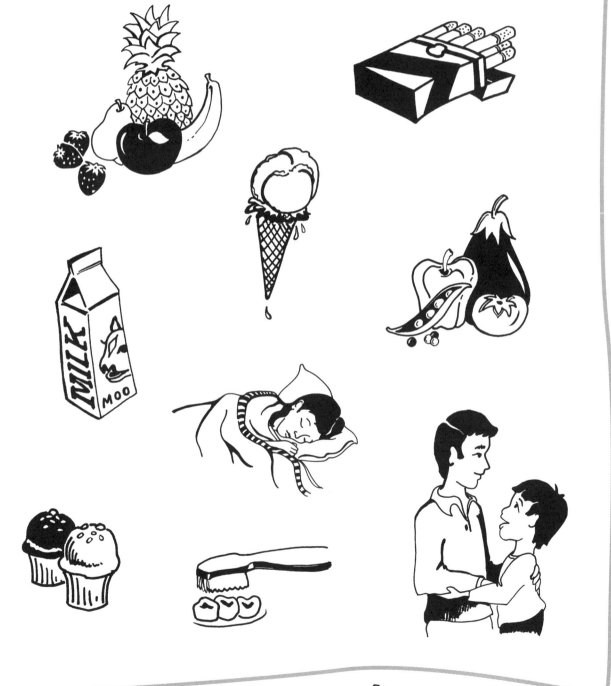

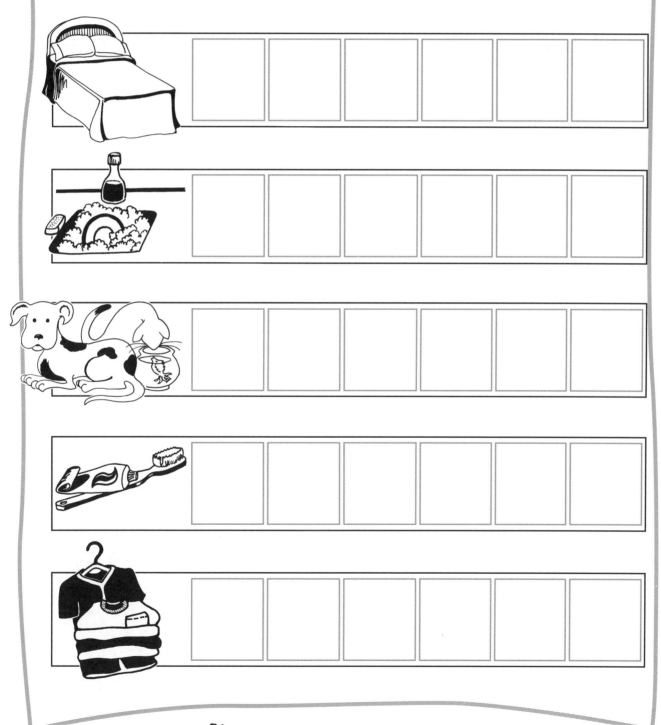

What Animal Am I?

Some Native Americans have a favorite animal that reminds them of something about themselves. What kind of animal would you be? Write a fable (or fairy tale) or draw a picture of the animal that is like you.

What animals are like other members of your family? Why?

Character Trace

Trace your hand in the space below. On each finger, write something that you like about yourself.

My Favorite Thing to Do

Draw a picture or write a story about something you are really good at doing. It could be your favorite thing to do.

Trophy Design

You get to award a trophy. Color the trophy and write a message on it for the person to whom you would give it.

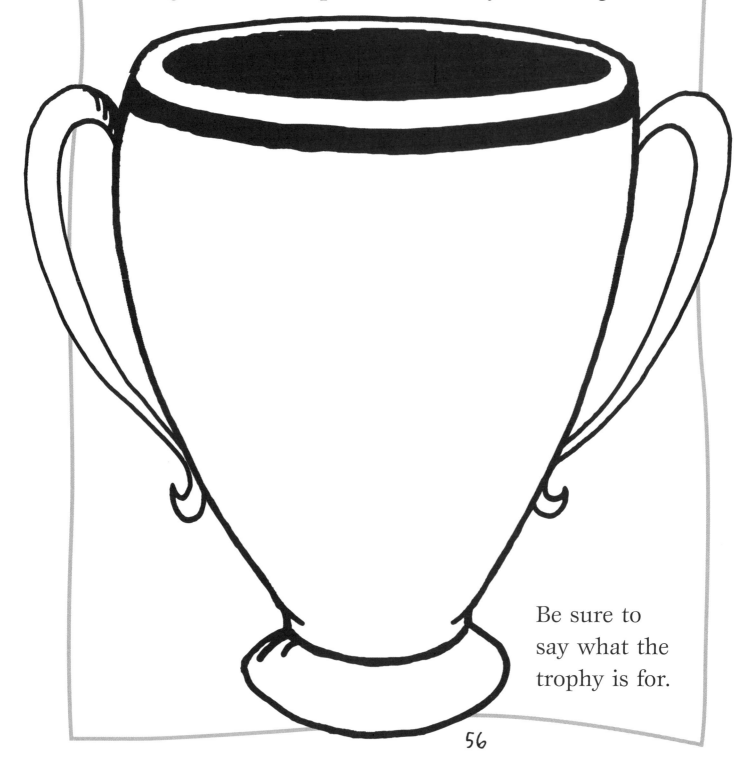

Be sure to say what the trophy is for.

YOU CAN HANDLE IT

People deal with worries in many different ways. Some people talk to a friend or family member. Others may write in a diary.

This part of your book will help you deal with your worries about the person you love who has cancer.

Where Are You Now?

Draw or write your answers to the questions below.

What has been the easiest thing about
_____'s cancer?

What has been the hardest thing?

What have you been most surprised about?

What do you want to know now?

What are you still worried about?

When the person you love goes to the hospital, how do you feel?

How will you feel when the cancer treatment is over?

Building Blocks of Helpers

Draw pictures or write the names of the people who help you with the things in the squares.

Someone you can talk to about the person you love who has cancer

Someone who can answer your questions

Someone who can fix something for you

Someone you can talk to about your feelings

Someone you can have fun with

Someone who can help you with your clothes, schoolwork, or sports

In the Laboratory

Pretend you are a scientist. What would you create in your laboratory to destroy cancer? Write a story or draw a picture.

Find Healing

Fill in the blanks to find the path to healing.

Clues

H 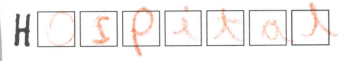 Place where doctors and nurses work

E 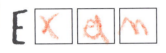 Another word for a test

A 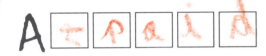 Another word for scared

L 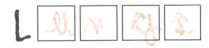 These are used to breathe

I 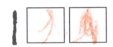 Another word for sick

N 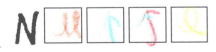 Person who works with doctors and is trained to care for people who are sick.

G 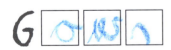 What you wear when you stay in the hospital

1) Hospital; 2) Exam; 3) Afraid; 4) Lungs; 5) Ill; 6) Nurse; 7) Gown.

Helping Out Coupon

Create a coupon for doing a chore. Cut it out and give the coupon to a special person that you would like to help.

COUPON!

SPECIAL OFFER FOR A SPECIAL PERSON

COUPON!

SPECIAL OFFER FOR A SPECIAL PERSON

©2003 American Cancer Society. All rights reserved. Copies of this page may be reproduced only for personal, educational, and/or noncommercial use by the reader.

COUPON!
WITH LOVE, FROM:

COUPON!
WITH LOVE, FROM:

Will It Come Back?

Everyone worries that the person they love might get cancer again. Write a story or draw a picture about your worries or fears about the cancer coming back.

Picture of the Future

Draw a picture of a wish you have for yourself and your family five years from now.

Scare It Away

Scarecrows scare birds away from gardens. Draw your own scarecrow.

What is it scaring away? _____

_____

_____

Screen-Saver Message

Many people put special messages or thoughts on their computer screens. Write a screen-saver message or draw a picture on the screen about cancer.

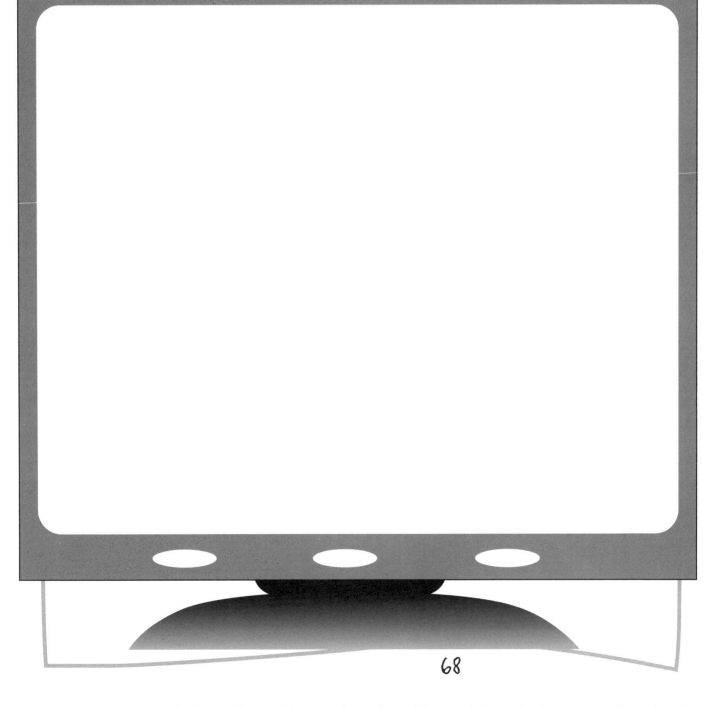

Hospital Bracelet

Special bracelets are given to patients who are in the hospital. Create a hospital bracelet to remind the person who has cancer that you love him or her. You may draw a picture or write get-well wishes. Cut it out and give it to your special someone.

70

Get Well Card

Cut along the solid lines. Fold the paper in half along the dotted line. Create a "Get Well" card to give to the person you love who has cancer.

To-Do List

Fill out a list of things you want to do with your loved one who has cancer when she or he feels better.

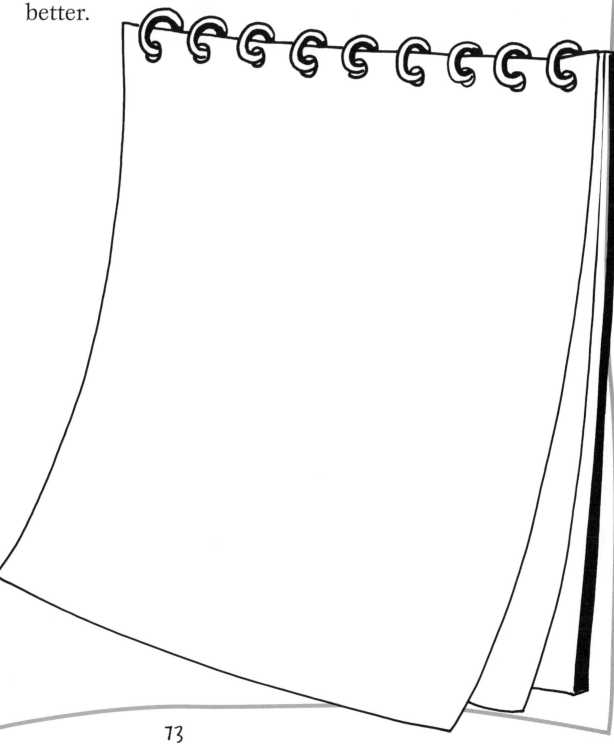

Laughter Is Good Medicine

Laughter can make you feel better. Write a story or draw a picture of something that made you laugh.

Thank You!

Write a note or letter of thanks for the special someone who takes care of the person you love who has cancer. You may cut out your note and give it to that person if you wish.

Thank You!

Happy Memories

Write or draw about happy memories you have of the person you love who is sick. Return to this page to remember these memories if you're feeling down.

Good Times

Draw a picture or write a story about a special day with your family. How did you feel then?

Welcome Home!

Your loved one is coming home! Design a "Welcome Home!" banner.

©2003 American Cancer Society. All rights reserved. Copies of this page may be reproduced only for personal, educational, and/or noncommercial use by the reader.